SCOLIOSIS DIET PLAN COOK BOOK

The Complete Scoliosis Diet Plan: Restorative Foods for Better Spinal Function

LARRY HERMAN

Table of Contents

Introduction.........................5

CHAPTER ONE 10

Definition and Types of Scoliosis 10

Causes and Risk Factors 15

CHAPTER TWO.........................21

Symptoms and Diagnosis........21

Importance of Diet in Managing Scoliosis 26

CHAPTER THREE 31

How Diet Affects Spinal Health 31

Designing a Scoliosis-Friendly Diet Plan 36

CHAPTER FOUR.........................42

Nutrients and Supplements ...42

Meal Planning for Scoliosis Patients 49

Implementing lifestyle modifications to manage scoliosis 56

Conclusion............................63

THE END................................67

Introduction

Scoliosis is a pathological disorder distinguished by an atypical bending of the vertebral column. Although nutrition alone cannot cure or reverse scoliosis, adhering to a healthy and balanced diet can help manage the illness and enhance overall well-being. It is crucial to acknowledge that there is no scientific evidence supporting the effectiveness of a specific "scoliosis diet," and any dietary suggestions should be consulted with healthcare professionals.

Below are some overarching factors to consider when it comes to diet and scoliosis:

• Consuming a diet that is abundant in vital nutrients, such as vitamins, minerals, and antioxidants, can promote general health. Foods such as fruits, vegetables, whole grains, lean proteins, and dairy products help enhance a comprehensive nutritional profile.

• Sufficient consumption of calcium and vitamin D is essential for preserving bone health. Given that scoliosis affects the spine, it may be advantageous to ensure an adequate intake of these nutrients. Excellent sources of calcium comprise dairy products, such as milk and cheese, as well as leafy green vegetables like spinach and kale. Additionally, fortified foods, which have been enriched with calcium, are also good sources of this essential mineral. Vitamin D is commonly acquired from exposure to sunlight and can also be found in fatty fish, fortified dairy products, and supplements.

• **Sustaining Optimal Weight:** Having an excessive amount of body weight has the potential to worsen the difficulties linked to scoliosis, since it adds extra pressure on the spine. Hence, it is crucial to uphold a healthy weight by adhering to a well-balanced diet and engaging in consistent physical exercise in order to promote overall well-being.

• Incorporating anti-inflammatory items into the diet may provide relief for persons with scoliosis who experience discomfort or pain. Omega-3 fatty acids, which are abundant in fatty fish, flaxseeds, and walnuts, as well as antioxidants found in fruits and vegetables, are believed to possess anti-inflammatory characteristics.

• **Water Intake:** Maintaining proper hydration is crucial for optimal health and can contribute to the preservation of muscle and joint flexibility. Optimal hydration promotes the body's inherent processes and potentially enhances overall well-being for those with scoliosis.

It is important to highlight that although these dietary considerations can promote overall health and well-being, they should not be seen as a substitute for medical interventions or other treatments advised by healthcare professionals. Individuals diagnosed with scoliosis should seek guidance from their healthcare team, which may consist of orthopedic doctors, physical therapists, and dietitians, in order to create a complete and tailored strategy for managing their disease.

CHAPTER ONE
Definition and Types of Scoliosis

Scoliosis is a pathological disorder distinguished by an atypical curvature of the spinal column. Scoliosis is a condition when the spine deviates from its natural curved shape and instead curves laterally. Curvature of the spine can manifest in many areas and result in issues such as pain, discomfort, and, in extreme instances, reduced organ function. Scoliosis can impact individuals across all age groups; however it frequently becomes apparent during phases of accelerated development, such as puberty.

Scoliosis can be categorized into various categories, which are determined by different criteria. The primary categories comprise:

1. Idiopathic Scoliosis: This is the predominant kind of scoliosis, characterized by an unknown etiology. Idiopathic scoliosis usually emerges throughout puberty, however it can manifest at any stage of life. It is additionally classified according to the age at which it begins:

• There are two types of idiopathic scoliosis that occur during different age ranges: infantile idiopathic scoliosis, which occurs in children aged 0-3 years, and juvenile idiopathic scoliosis, which occurs in children aged 4-10 years.

• Adolescent idiopathic scoliosis occurs in individuals between the ages of 11 and 18.

2. Congenital Scoliosis: Congenital scoliosis is a condition that is present from birth and occurs due to anomalies in the construction of the spine during fetal development. This form of scoliosis is frequently linked to additional congenital abnormalities.

3. Neuromuscular scoliosis is a condition resulting from abnormalities that impact the muscles or nerves, causing an uneven distribution of muscle strength and curvature of the spine. Neuromuscular scoliosis can be caused by conditions such as cerebral palsy, muscular dystrophy, or spinal cord injury.

4. Degenerative Scoliosis, sometimes referred to as adult-onset scoliosis, is a condition that occurs in adulthood as a result of the gradual deterioration of the spine. It is commonly linked to the process of getting older and medical disorders like osteoarthritis.

Functional scoliosis:

The user's text is simply "o".Functional scoliosis is characterized by the presence of a curved spine, despite the spine being physically normal. Non-spinal causes, such as muscular imbalances, differences in leg length, or postural habits, are usually responsible for this form of scoliosis.

• The severity of scoliosis is commonly evaluated by the extent of curvature in the spinal column, typically determined with X-ray imaging. Less severe cases may not necessitate substantial treatment, however more severe cases may entail the use of braces, physical therapy, or, in extreme instances, surgical intervention to rectify the curvature.

Prompt identification and timely management are essential for properly managing scoliosis. Individuals who have concerns about the health of their spine should seek assessment from a healthcare professional, specifically orthopedic specialists or spine specialists.

Causes and Risk Factors

The exact cause of idiopathic scoliosis, which is the most common type, remains unknown. However, there are various factors that are believed to contribute to the development of scoliosis, and these can vary depending on the type of scoliosis. Here are some general causes and risk factors associated with scoliosis:

Idiopathic Scoliosis:

- **Genetics:** There is evidence to suggest a genetic component to idiopathic scoliosis. Individuals with a family history of scoliosis are at a higher risk of developing the condition.

• **Growth Spurts:** The onset of scoliosis often coincides with growth spurts during adolescence. Rapid growth may contribute to the development or progression of the curvature.

Congenital Scoliosis:

• Fetal Development Issues: Congenital scoliosis is caused by abnormalities in the formation of the spine during fetal development. Factors such as improper vertebral formation or segmentation can lead to congenital scoliosis.

Neuromuscular Scoliosis:

• Disorders affecting muscles and nerves: Conditions such as cerebral palsy, muscular dystrophy, spinal cord injuries, or neurofibromatosis can result in imbalances in muscle strength, leading to the development of scoliosis.

Degenerative Scoliosis:

• Aging: As people age, the spinal discs may degenerate, leading to changes in the structure and stability of the spine. This can contribute to the development of scoliosis in adulthood.

Functional Scoliosis:

• Muscle Imbalances: Muscular imbalances or irregularities, leg length discrepancies, and poor posture can contribute to functional scoliosis. These factors may cause the spine to appear curved, even though its structure is normal.

Risk factors for scoliosis include:

• **Age and Gender:** Adolescent idiopathic scoliosis is most commonly diagnosed during the growth spurt that occurs just before puberty. Girls are more likely than boys to have progressive idiopathic scoliosis, especially in severe cases.

• **Family History:** A family history of scoliosis increases the likelihood of an individual developing the condition. Genetic factors play a role in predisposing some individuals to scoliosis.

- **Other Medical Conditions:** Certain neuromuscular and connective tissue disorders, such as Marfan syndrome, can increase the risk of scoliosis.

- **Trauma or Injury:** While not a common cause, some cases of scoliosis may result from trauma or injury to the spine.

It's important to note that many cases of scoliosis are mild and may not cause significant health issues. Regular check-ups, especially during periods of rapid growth, can help detect scoliosis early, allowing for timely intervention and management. Individuals with concerns about their spinal health should consult with healthcare professionals, particularly orthopedic specialists or spine specialists, for proper evaluation and guidance.

CHAPTER TWO
Symptoms and Diagnosis

Symptoms of scoliosis can vary depending on the severity of the spinal curvature. In mild cases, individuals may not experience noticeable symptoms, while more severe cases can lead to visible changes in posture and potential health issues. Common signs and symptoms of scoliosis include:

• **Uneven Shoulders or Hips:** One shoulder or hip may appear higher than the other.

• **Uneven Waist:** The waistline may be uneven or tilted.

• **Prominent Shoulder Blade:** One shoulder blade may be more prominent or stick out compared to the other.

• **Asymmetric Appearance:** The spine may appear twisted or rotated, causing an asymmetrical appearance of the back.

• **Clothing Fit Changes:** Clothes may not hang evenly, and there may be a noticeable difference in the fit on one side of the body.

• **Back Pain or Discomfort:** Some individuals with scoliosis may experience back pain or discomfort, especially as the curvature progresses.

• **Limited Range of Motion:** In severe cases, scoliosis can lead to a decreased range of motion in the spine.

• Diagnosis of scoliosis typically involves a combination of medical history, physical examination, and imaging studies. Healthcare professionals, particularly orthopedic specialists or spine specialists, may perform the following:

• **Physical Examination:** The healthcare provider will assess the individual's posture, gait, and spinal alignment. They may ask the person to bend forward at the waist to check for asymmetry, rib hump, or other signs of scoliosis.

• **Adam's Forward Bend Test:** During this test, the individual is asked to bend forward at the waist, allowing the healthcare provider to observe any spinal curvature.

• **Imaging Studies:** X-rays are commonly used to confirm the diagnosis and provide detailed images of the spine. X-rays help measure the degree of curvature and determine the type of scoliosis.

• **MRI or CT Scan:** In some cases, especially when evaluating congenital or neuromuscular scoliosis, additional imaging studies like magnetic resonance imaging (MRI) or computed tomography (CT) scans may be recommended to assess the spinal structures more thoroughly.

Once diagnosed, the healthcare team will determine the appropriate course of action based on factors such as the degree of curvature, the type of scoliosis, and the individual's age. Treatment options may include observation, bracing, physical therapy, or, in severe cases, surgery. Regular monitoring is essential to track the progression of scoliosis and adjust the treatment plan as needed. Early detection and intervention play a crucial role in managing scoliosis effectively. Individuals with concerns about their spinal health should seek evaluation from qualified healthcare professionals.

Importance of Diet in Managing Scoliosis

While diet alone cannot cure or directly treat scoliosis, maintaining a healthy and well-balanced diet is important for overall health and may play a supportive role in managing the condition. Here are some ways in which diet can be beneficial for individuals with scoliosis:

- **Bone Health:** Adequate intake of calcium and vitamin D is crucial for maintaining bone health. Since scoliosis involves the spine, ensuring proper bone density is important. Calcium-rich foods, such as dairy products, leafy green vegetables, and fortified foods, contribute to bone strength. Vitamin D, obtained through sunlight exposure and certain foods like fatty fish and fortified dairy products, helps the body absorb calcium.

- **Muscle and Tissue Health:** A well-balanced diet provides essential nutrients that support muscle and tissue health. Protein, found in sources like lean meats, poultry, fish, legumes, and dairy products, is important for muscle maintenance and repair.

- **Anti-Inflammatory Foods:** Some individuals with scoliosis may experience discomfort or pain. Including anti-inflammatory foods in the diet, such as those rich in omega-3 fatty acids (found in fatty fish, flaxseeds, and walnuts) and antioxidants (found in fruits and vegetables), may help manage inflammation and contribute to overall comfort.

- **Maintaining a Healthy Weight:** Excess body weight can potentially exacerbate the challenges associated with scoliosis by placing additional strain on the spine. Adopting a balanced diet and engaging in regular physical activity can contribute to maintaining a healthy weight.

- **Hydration:** Staying well-hydrated is important for overall health and can help maintain the flexibility of muscles and joints. Proper hydration supports the body's natural functions and may contribute to overall comfort for individuals with scoliosis.

It's essential to note that while a healthy diet is beneficial, it does not replace medical interventions or other treatments recommended by healthcare professionals. The primary focus of scoliosis management often involves monitoring the curvature, providing physical therapy, using braces if necessary, and, in severe cases, considering surgical options.

Individuals with scoliosis should work closely with their healthcare team, including orthopedic specialists, physical therapists, and nutritionists, to develop a comprehensive approach tailored to their specific needs. Nutrition recommendations may vary based on the individual's overall health, the type and severity of scoliosis, and any other underlying medical conditions. Always consult with healthcare professionals for personalized advice and guidance.

CHAPTER THREE
How Diet Affects Spinal Health

Nutrition plays a vital role in promoting general well-being, and this also applies to the health of the spine. There are multiple ways in which nutrition can impact and contribute to the overall health of the spine:

Nutrient Intake for B one Health:

• Adequate intake of essential nutrients, such as calcium and vitamin D, is crucial for maintaining bone health. The spine is a key component of the skeletal system, and strong, healthy bones are essential for supporting the spine's structure. Calcium-rich foods (dairy products, leafy green vegetables) and vitamin D (fatty fish, fortified dairy products, sunlight exposure) are important for bone density.

Protein for Muscle Support:

• Protein is essential for muscle maintenance, repair, and overall support. The muscles surrounding the spine play a vital role in providing stability and preventing issues related to spinal alignment. Sources of protein include lean meats, poultry, fish, legumes, and dairy products.

Omega-3 Fatty Acids for Anti-Inflammatory Effects:

• Omega-3 fatty acids, found in fatty fish (such as salmon and mackerel), flaxseeds, and walnuts, have anti-inflammatory properties. Inflammation can contribute to pain and discomfort associated with various spinal conditions. Including omega-3-rich foods in the diet may help manage inflammation and promote spinal health.

Antioxidants for Tissue Health:

• Fruits and vegetables, rich in antioxidants, play a role in protecting tissues from oxidative stress. Oxidative stress can contribute to the breakdown of tissues, and maintaining a diet high in antioxidants supports overall tissue health, including that of the spinal structures.

Maintaining a Healthy Weight:

• Excess body weight can place additional stress on the spine, leading to issues such as back pain and an increased risk of musculoskeletal conditions. A balanced diet, combined with regular physical activity, can help individuals maintain a healthy weight and reduce the burden on the spine.

Hydration for Joint Health:

• Staying well-hydrated is essential for the health of intervertebral discs, which act as cushions between the vertebrae in the spine. Proper hydration helps maintain the elasticity and shock-absorbing properties of these discs, contributing to joint health.

Balanced Nutrition for Overall Wellness:

• A well-balanced diet provides the body with the necessary nutrients for overall health and wellness. This includes vitamins, minerals, and other essential components that support the body's natural functions, including those related to the spine.

While diet is important for spinal health, it's crucial to recognize that it is just one aspect of overall well-being. Specific spinal conditions may require targeted interventions, such as physical therapy, medications, or surgical procedures. Individuals with spinal concerns or conditions should consult with healthcare professionals, including orthopedic specialists or spine specialists, for comprehensive evaluation and guidance tailored to their specific needs.

Designing a Scoliosis-Friendly Diet Plan

Creating a dietary regimen for individuals with scoliosis entails emphasizing the consumption of nourishing foods that promote general well-being, enhance bone integrity, and optimize muscular performance. Although there is no specific diet designed exclusively for scoliosis, including essential nutrients in your diet can be advantageous. Below is a comprehensive outline for a diet plan that is suitable for those with scoliosis:

1. Foods high in calcium: Incorporate dairy products (milk, yogurt, cheese), leafy green vegetables (kale, broccoli), and fortified foods into your diet to guarantee a sufficient intake of calcium, which promotes bone health.

2. Sources of Vitamin D: Obtain vitamin D by exposing yourself to sunlight and incorporating foods such as fatty fish (salmon, mackerel), fortified dairy products, and egg yolks into your diet.

3. Choose lean sources of protein such as poultry, fish, lean cuts of meat, lentils, and tofu. Protein plays a vital role in the preservation and restoration of muscles.

4. Omega-3 Fatty Acids: Include fatty fish (such as salmon and mackerel), flaxseeds, chia seeds, and walnuts in your diet to obtain anti-inflammatory omega-3 fatty acids.

5. Consume a diverse range of colored fruits and vegetables to ensure a wide array of antioxidants, which promote tissue health. Optimal selections include berries, citrus fruits, spinach, and bell peppers.

6. Opt for whole grains like brown rice, quinoa, whole wheat bread, and oats to obtain fiber, vitamins, and minerals that contribute to general health.

7. **Hydration:** Ensure optimal hydration by consuming ample amounts of water. Optimal hydration is crucial for preserving the well-being of intervertebral discs.

8. Reduce the consumption of processed meals, sugary drinks, and excessive quantities of refined carbs. These foods have the potential to cause inflammation and lead to an increase in body weight.

9. Implement portion management as a means of managing weight and promoting overall health. Obesity can exert extra pressure on the spinal column.

10. Consistent Meals: Strive for consistent, well-balanced meals to ensure a consistent flow of nutrients throughout the day.

11. When creating a diet plan, it is crucial to take into account an individual's specific dietary restrictions, preferences, or underlying health conditions in order to customize the plan accordingly. Seek guidance from a healthcare practitioner or a qualified dietician for individualized recommendations.

Please note that this broad guidance does not serve as a replacement for expert medical advice. Individuals diagnosed with scoliosis should collaborate closely with healthcare professionals, such as orthopedic doctors and nutritionists, to ensure that their food regimen is tailored to their individual health requirements and compliments their entire treatment plan. Individuals may need to regularly examine and make adjustments to their diet based on their specific health issues and the outcomes of their therapy.

CHAPTER FOUR
Nutrients and Supplements

While a well-balanced diet is the primary source of essential nutrients, some individuals, including those with scoliosis, may consider supplements to ensure they meet their nutritional needs. It's important to note that dietary supplements should be used under the guidance of healthcare professionals, as excessive intake of certain nutrients can have adverse effects. Here are some nutrients and supplements that may be relevant to individuals with scoliosis:

Calcium:

- Essential for bone health, calcium is crucial for individuals with scoliosis. Dairy products, leafy green vegetables, and fortified foods are good dietary sources. If dietary intake is insufficient, calcium supplements may be considered, but their use should be supervised by a healthcare provider.

Vitamin D:

- Vitamin D is important for calcium absorption and bone health. Exposure to sunlight is a natural source, and dietary sources include fatty fish and fortified dairy products. In some cases, vitamin D supplements may be recommended, especially for individuals with limited sun exposure or difficulty obtaining sufficient vitamin D through food.

Omega-3 Fatty Acids:

- Omega-3 fatty acids have anti-inflammatory properties. Fatty fish (salmon, mackerel), flaxseeds, and walnuts are dietary sources. If these foods are not regularly consumed, omega-3 supplements such as fish oil capsules may be considered, but again, consultation with a healthcare professional is advised.

Multivitamins:

- A multivitamin may be recommended to fill potential nutritional gaps. However, relying on a balanced diet is generally preferred over relying solely on supplements.

Protein:

- Protein is essential for muscle maintenance and repair. Dietary sources include lean meats, poultry, fish, legumes, and tofu. Protein supplements are generally not necessary if a well-rounded diet is maintained.

Magnesium:

- Magnesium is involved in bone health and muscle function. Dietary sources include nuts, seeds, whole grains, and green leafy vegetables. Magnesium supplements may be considered if there is a deficiency, but it's important to be monitored by healthcare professionals.

Vitamin K:

- Vitamin K is important for bone health, and green leafy vegetables are good dietary sources. Individuals taking blood-thinning medications should consult with their healthcare provider before taking vitamin K supplements.

Iron:

- Iron is important for overall health and oxygen transport in the blood. While some individuals with scoliosis may have iron deficiency, excessive iron intake can be harmful. Iron supplements should be taken only under the guidance of healthcare professionals.

It's crucial to emphasize that supplements should not be used as a substitute for a healthy and balanced diet. Nutrient needs can vary among individuals, and excessive intake of certain vitamins and minerals can have adverse effects. Before starting any supplementation, individuals with scoliosis should consult with healthcare professionals, including a registered dietitian or a healthcare provider, to assess their specific nutritional needs and determine the appropriate supplements, if any. Regular monitoring and adjustment of supplements may be necessary based on individual health conditions and treatment outcomes.

Meal Planning for Scoliosis Patients

Meal planning for individuals with scoliosis should focus on a balanced and nutrient-rich diet to support overall health, bone strength, and muscle function. Here's a sample meal plan that incorporates key nutrients for individuals with scoliosis:

Breakfast:

Option 1: Oatmeal with Berries and Nuts

- **Ingredients:** Rolled oats, water or milk, mixed berries (blueberries, strawberries), chopped nuts (walnuts or almonds), a drizzle of honey.

- **Benefits:** Oats provide fiber and whole grains, berries offer antioxidants, and nuts provide omega-3 fatty acids.

Option 2: Greek Yogurt Parfait

- **Ingredients:** Greek yogurt, granola, sliced bananas, and a sprinkle of chia seeds.
- **Benefits:** Greek yogurt is a good source of protein and calcium, while granola and chia seeds add fiber and nutrients.

Mid-Morning Snack:

Fresh Fruit and Nut Mix

- **Ingredients:** Apple slices, grapes, and a small handful of mixed nuts (almonds, walnuts).
- **Benefits:** Provides additional vitamins, antioxidants, and healthy fats.

Lunch:

Grilled Salmon Salad

- **Ingredients:** Grilled salmon, mixed greens, cherry tomatoes, cucumber, quinoa, and a light vinaigrette dressing.
- **Benefits:** Salmon is rich in omega-3 fatty acids, while the salad provides a variety of vitamins and minerals.

Afternoon Snack:

Carrot and Hummus

- **Ingredients:** Carrot sticks with a side of hummus.
- **Benefits:** Carrots supply beta-carotene, and hummus offers protein and healthy fats.

Dinner:

Chicken Stir-Fry with Vegetables

- **Ingredients:** Grilled chicken breast, stir-fried broccoli, bell peppers, carrots, and brown rice.
- **Benefits:** Lean protein from chicken, a variety of colorful

vegetables, and whole grains from brown rice.

Evening Snack:

Greek Yogurt with a Dash of Cinnamon

- **Ingredients**: Greek yogurt with a sprinkle of cinnamon.
- **Benefits:** Greek yogurt provides additional protein and calcium.

Hydration:

- Throughout the day, ensure adequate water intake. Herbal teas or infused water with slices of citrus fruits can be refreshing and hydrating.

Considerations:

Portion Control:

- Pay attention to portion sizes to maintain a healthy weight and prevent excess stress on the spine.

Limit Processed Foods and Sugary Drinks:

- Minimize the intake of processed foods and sugary beverages, as they may contribute to inflammation and weight gain.

Individualized Adjustments:

- Depending on individual dietary preferences, allergies, or specific nutritional needs, adjust the meal plan accordingly.

Consultation with Healthcare Professionals:

- Always consult with healthcare professionals, including a registered dietitian or a healthcare provider, to tailor the meal plan to individual health requirements.

This sample meal plan provides a variety of nutrients, including calcium, vitamin D, omega-3 fatty acids, protein, and antioxidants. It serves as a general guide, and individuals with scoliosis should work closely with healthcare professionals to create a personalized meal plan that aligns with their specific health needs and complements their overall treatment plan.

Implementing lifestyle modifications to manage scoliosis

The management of scoliosis typically entails a blend of lifestyle modifications, medicinal therapies, and, occasionally, surgical operations. Below are lifestyle modifications that can be advantageous for individuals with scoliosis:

1. Consistent Physical Activity: Participate in regular exercise to enhance flexibility, muscular strength, and overall well-being of the spine.

Engaging in activities such as swimming, yoga, and Pilates can yield significant advantages. Nevertheless, it is crucial to get guidance from healthcare experts, such as physical therapists, in order to identify the most appropriate workouts for specific requirements.

2. Sustain an Optimal Body Mass: Ensure that your body mass remains within a healthy range in order to minimize the strain on the spine. Excessive body weight can lead to additional strain on the spine and potentially worsen scoliosis. Following a well-rounded diet and engaging in consistent physical activity can assist in attaining and sustaining a healthy body weight.

3. Maintaining Posture Awareness: Be mindful of your posture throughout everyday tasks, such as sitting, standing, or walking. Adhering to proper posture can effectively reduce strain on the spinal column. It is also worth considering making ergonomic changes to desks and chairs.

4. Consistent Surveillance: Continuously observe any alterations in the curvature of the spine. Regular consultations with medical professionals, including orthopedic specialists, are crucial for monitoring the advancement of scoliosis and implementing any required modifications to the treatment regimen.

5. Adaptive equipment and assistive devices can be beneficial for those with mobility issues due to scoliosis. These tools can enhance everyday functioning and alleviate stress on the spine.

6. Engage in physical therapy sessions to acquire knowledge about exercises and strategies that specifically address scoliosis. Physical therapists are able to create individualized treatment plans to target muscle imbalances and improve the stability of the spine.

7. Orthopedic bracing is a recommended treatment for persons with moderate scoliosis. It helps prevent the curvature from worsening, particularly during periods of rapid growth in adolescence. Adherence to the recommended brace is crucial for its efficacy.

8. Pain Management Techniques: Utilize pain management techniques, such as thermotherapy or cryotherapy, manual manipulation, and mindfulness exercises, to mitigate the discomfort associated with scoliosis. Healthcare providers may provide recommendations on the usage of over-the-counter pain medications.

9. Psychological Support: Obtain psychological support, particularly for adolescents grappling with body image issues associated with scoliosis. assistance groups or counseling can offer individuals emotional assistance and effective coping mechanisms.

10. Education and Self-Care: Acquire knowledge about scoliosis and its treatment. Gaining comprehension of the condition enables patients to actively engage in their own healthcare. Engage in self-care activities, such as employing stress management strategies, in order to enhance one's overall state of well-being.

Collaboration with a healthcare team, consisting of orthopedic doctors, physical therapists, and other pertinent professionals, is imperative for persons with scoliosis. Customized treatment programs are frequently designed to address the unique condition of each individual, and lifestyle modifications are incorporated alongside medical interventions to provide the most effective management of scoliosis. Frequent communication with healthcare providers guarantees that the treatment plan is modified as necessary, taking into account the individual's progress and specific health requirements.

Conclusion

To summarize, the management of scoliosis requires a comprehensive approach that integrates medical therapies, adjustments to one's lifestyle, and continuous monitoring. Although there is no designated "scoliosis diet," adhering to a well-balanced and nutrient-dense diet can enhance general health, bolster bone integrity, and optimize muscular performance. Ensuring sufficient consumption of calcium, vitamin D, omega-3 fatty acids, and other crucial minerals is imperative.

- Essential components of scoliosis care include adopting a healthy lifestyle, which involves engaging in regular physical activity, maintaining an optimal body weight, practicing proper posture, and actively participating in physical therapy. Consistent surveillance by medical practitioners, such as orthopedic experts and physical therapists, facilitates the monitoring of scoliosis advancement and enables modifications to the treatment regimen as necessary.

• Individuals diagnosed with scoliosis should take an active role in managing their illness, including seeking psychological assistance as necessary and staying well-informed about the condition. Engaging in collaboration with a healthcare team guarantees the development of a customized treatment plan that effectively targets the unique requirements of every individual.

The primary objective of scoliosis care is to optimize general health, alleviate discomfort, and halt the advancement of the spine curvature. Through the integration of medical competence and the adoption of healthy lifestyle choices, persons diagnosed with scoliosis can effectively pursue active and gratifying lifestyles. Seeking guidance from healthcare specialists is crucial for accurate assessment, diagnosis, and the formulation of a tailored and efficient treatment strategy if you or someone you are acquainted with is affected by scoliosis.

THE END

www.ingramcontent.com/pod-product-compliance
Lightning Source LLC
Chambersburg PA
CBHW061308250726
48653CB00002B/843